This Therapy Journal belongs to:

. . . .

Therapy Journal
The mental health journal
that makes the most of your therapy sessions

3rd Edition - December 2021

@adaytoremember_journals
adaytoremember.journals@gmail.com

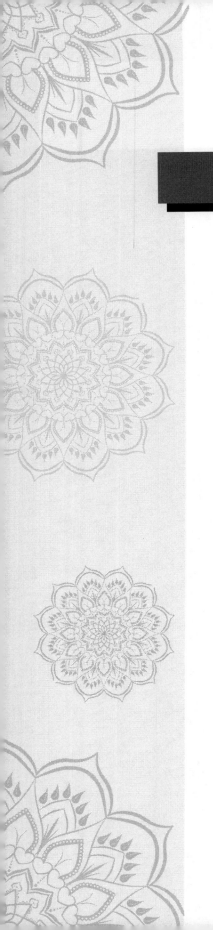

INDEX

3 OUR THANK YOU NOTE TO YOU

4 IMPORTANT INFORMATION

5 CRISIS RESOURCES CONTACT

6 INTRODUCTION

7-8 HOW TO USE YOUR JOURNAL

9-10 HOW TO GET THE MOST OUT OF YOUR THERAPY SESSIONS

11-13 THERAPY SESSIONS SCHEDULE

14 THERAPY GOALS

15-16 THERAPY TOOLS I LEARNED

17-77 THERAPY SESSION NOTES PAGES

78-97 ADDITIONAL NOTES PAGES

98-100 GET TO KNOW OUR JOURNALS & JOIN OUR TEAM!

Before you get started we'd like to introduce ourselves
and THANK YOU *for buying this journal!*

We are 2 high school friends just starting a journey of entrepreneurship.
(We're now "grown ups", moms; Carla is based in the USA, and Milena in Brazil).

We are challenging ourselves to create 52 journals this year, ~1 per week!
We are so grateful for your support so far, and we invite you to follow our journey.

Our promise: to make EVERY *customer happy*

We hope this journal will help you discover the benefits of therapy by making it an easier
and more organized process. We really believe that it will help bring improvements
to your life and even to those around you.

But if for any reason you are not satisfied with your journal, please contact us directly;
we will do our best to make you happy!

Your REVIEW *means a lot to us!*

And especially if you like this journal, would you please give us a couple minutes of your time
and write a review on Amazon?

This journal is now on its 3rd edition (we are improving it based on feedback).
Our goal for it is to reach 100 reviews on Amazon, which will give it more visibility and credibility.
We are at 71 reviews now (Amazon US website), so each new one makes a BIG difference.

Your honest review is a big encouragement for us, new creators and sellers, to keep going.
And it helps other people find our product, too!

(To leave a review go to the product page on Amazon, scroll down and select
"Write a customer review")

Let's be friends! - CONNECT *and* SHARE *with us*

If you would like to be part of our "launch team" to receive free samples of future journal
concepts, or if you'd like to share your journal ideas, comments or suggestions,
(or even complaints!) please connect with us & reach out:

 Instagram: @adaytoremember_journals
Amazon: follow "A Day to Remember Journals"
or email us at: adaytoremember.journals@gmail.com.

And please "tag us" on Instagram when you post about your experiences!
WE WOULD ♡ TO BE PART OF YOUR JOURNEY
the same way we feel that you are a BIG part of ours!

xoxo, Carla and Milena

Important Information

PATIENT INFORMATION:

Name:

Phone:

E-mail:

THERAPIST #1 INFORMATION:

Name:

Phone:

E-mail:

THERAPIST #2 INFORMATION:

Name:

Phone:

E-mail:

THERAPIST #3 INFORMATION:

Name:

Phone:

E-mail:

Crisis Resources Contacts

USA CRISIS RESOURCES:

USA Suicide Prevention Lifeline: Call 1-800-273 -8255
The National Suicide Prevention Lifeline is a national network of local crisis centers that provides free and confidential emotional support to people in suicidal crisis or emotional distress 24 hours a day, 7 days a week

Crisis Text Line: Text MHA to 741741
You'll be connected to a trained Crisis Counselor.
Crisis Text Line provides free, text-based support 24/7

Youthline: Text teen2teen to 839863 or Call (877)968-8491
A free 24-hour crisis, support, and helpline for youth. Talk to a teen volunteer daily from 4pm-10pm PST (and by adults at all other times!)

Hotline for LGBTQ Youth (The Trevor project): Call 1-866-488-7386 or text START to 678678.
A national 24-hour, toll free confidential suicide hotline for LGBTQ youth

LOCAL HELP CENTERS:
Write below where you can find help in your neighborhood or country, if you're outside of the USA

Name:

Phone   Hours:

Description (eg. Teen support):

Name:

Phone   Hours:

Description (eg. Teen support):

Name:

Phone   Hours:

Description (eg. Teen support):

Name:

Phone   Hours:

Description (eg. Teen support):

Introduction

For a long time I was resistant to the idea of "going to therapy".
I didn't believe that I needed to see a therapist, and I thought doing so would be a waste of my time.

But when you are struggling with a situation, sometimes you just have to try everything to overcome it. So I gave therapy a chance, and it changed me, it changed my life. (Thank you to my wonderful therapists Eva and Melissa!).

Now, after about 3 years of therapy, I wish I had documented highlights of my sessions, and had a timeline of my transformation.

I love to take notes, and I often did so during my sessions, but the notes were spread over many notebooks along with other unrelated information, so they are hard to retrieve now.

To solve this "problem" I created this Therapy Journal, which I myself use. It's been very handy to me, and I hope that it will be useful for you too! (I'd be so happy if you leave us a honest review on Amazon or send us a message - via Instagram or email - letting us know what you think of it!)

If you have ideas on how to make it better, let us know, too. We plan to update it regularly based on feedback received.

We hope that your healing will happen faster, and in a more intentional way with the help of this journal.

We trust that your self confidence will grow, and that you will find true happiness again, as I did myself.

Good Luck!

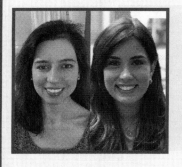

Hello! We are Carla and Mila, two best friends passionate about journaling and mental health. We have attended therapy for years and we know the benefits that it can bring to our lives. We also know that writing and reflecting on the sessions can bring us organization, encouragement and intentionality.

This journal was created from a patient point of view and it is meant to be a simple, practical and a useful tool for therapy patients.

We encourage you to fill the pages on this journal with your sessions notes, and to keep it also as a way to celebrate the progress that you will make over time.

<u>How to use this</u> Journal - Part 1

** How to get the most out of Therapy Sessions **

Read this section to find some guidance on how to make the most of this investment in yourself: your therapy sessions.
The information on this section talks about how to prepare for each therapy session, how to behave during the sessions, and more.

** Therapy Sessions Schedule **

Use this space to plan for your sessions in an organized way. Gradually fill in the date & time of the sessions, along with the name of your therapist and his/her contacts, address and/or some short note that you need to easily remember.

** Therapy Goals **

Here we encourage you to write your "big picture goals", those that you will be discussing over several therapy sessions. For example:
- improve a relationship / not allow a bad relationship to affect all areas of your life, or
- overcome drug addiction/depression, and so on.

We encourage you to write a date when that goal was established, and to also list some actions / things that could help - eg. exercising and reconnecting with friends.

** Therapy Tools I learned **

Therapy tools can help you throughout your journey.
Whenever you learn a tool capture it on this page so that you can easily refer back to it when you need it.

You may first write about the tool on the "insights page" of a therapy session (eg. when you learn about it from your therapist). But as soon as you have a feeling that a tool could help you in many occasions, you should also write the information on the "tools pages" for easy reference.

How to use this Journal - Part 2

** Therapy session notes pages **

- Pre and Post Session Tracker: Quickly mark how you feel before and at the end of each session - eg. how do you feel emotionally? How helpful the session was?

- Topic(s) I want to discuss or goal(s) my therapist had for the session: To get the most out of your sessions, help your therapist by coming prepared with your most pressing needs/questions. So before each of your therapy sessions, write down what you plan to talk about with or ask your therapist. Reflect about how this is affecting your life, and ways you may have tried to overcome the situation already.

If you don't have a clear goal in mind for the session, accept the suggestion from your therapist, and capture it on your journal.

- Notes from session: During your discussion with the therapist, or as soon as possible afterwards, write down your the main comments, insights and takeaways from the session.

Do not forget to write about **possible actions and follow ups!** And look back on these notes between sessions to see and sustain your progress.

- Things to remember: To conclude each of these pages, write down the main things that you want to remember from that day / therapy session.

** Additional Notes pages **

Every time you have a thought or idea that you believe will be an important one to remember and go back to over time, write it down in the "Additional Notes pages".

Capture the date and other relevant aspects related to your thought or idea.

Let's get started!

How to get the most out of Therapy Sessions?

CHOOSE YOUR THERAPIST CAREFULLY

It's a good idea to take time to carefully choose your therapist. Research different types of therapists and approaches and when you start, assess how comfortable you feel talking to him/her.

FIND THE RIGHT TIME

Schedule and reserve the necessary space of time for your session. Don't try to fit it in the middle of your school classes or your work meetings. You need time and space to process and reflect around the therapy hour.

SET GOALS FOR YOUR THERAPY

It's important to establish goals for positive change with your therapist , so that you'll be better able to track your progress and stay motivated. They can be simple goals, such as feeling happier or more energized. Think about what are the right goals for you and go for them.

BE OPEN IN YOUR SESSIONS: SAY WHATEVER YOU WANT

When in session, say whatever you want, because doing so is what really leads to progress. Trust is important and you need to be the most unfiltered version of yourself. (That said, of course, we should always be respectful with the therapist).

VIEW THERAPY AS A COLLABORATION

Therapy is an interactive process. Express your needs, ask questions, and discuss what you'd like to share during each session. But the therapist certainly wants to help you, so accept his/her guidance, too - even when it may feel a bit uncomfortable.

DO THE WORK BEFORE & AFTER THE SESSIONS

Take you thoughts and takeaways of your sessions beyond the session itself. Think about them whenever you can. This process, as the act of writing on this journal will help you reflect and prepare for the next sessions.

TAKE SOME MINUTES BEFORE THE SESSION TO RELAX

Take a few minutes before the session to calm down, relax and get in the mood. For instance, you may listen to calm music while you read on this journal reminders of the topics you want to talk about during the session. This will help you organize your thoughts about how you are going to approach the session and make the most of it.

KEEP PAPER & PEN HANDY DURING YOUR SESSIONS

It may be this journal or another paper, but you will probably want and we strongly encourage that you write down your insights.

HAVE AN AUTHENTIC CONNECTION WITH YOUR THERAPIST

The connection between a therapist and a person in therapy is very important. To accomplish this, be direct with your therapist. This will help your therapist help you, and beyond that, it will also help you get comfortable with parts of yourself that you may tend to hide. Remember you shouldn't just "show up" to therapy; you need to "open up",too.

SET BOUNDARIES WITH PEOPLE AROUND YOU

It's important not to share details of your sessions with people who you don't trust or with whom you don't feel safe around.
Set boundaries so you don't have to deal with gossip and intrusive people.

CHANGE THERAPIST, IF YOU NEED

If you feel that even after trying it for a while, you're really not happy with how it's going, you may want to consider talking to your therapist about any issues you're having with him/her, and maybe even consider changing your therapist.

ENJOY YOUR PROCESS

Therapy can be amazing.

Take your time and enjoy each session and progress.

Celebrate small wins.

Enjoy the journey!

Therapy Sessions Schedule

	DATE/TIME	THERAPIST	THERAPIST CONTACT	ADDRESS/ NOTE
SESSION 1	Nov 15, 2021	Sandra Jones	917 689 xxxx	*Example* Virtual session; use link on email (or 89 Park Ave)
SESSION 2				
SESSION 3				
SESSION 4				
SESSION 5				
SESSION 6				
SESSION 7				
SESSION 8				
SESSION 9				

	DATE/TIME	THERAPIST	THERAPIST CONTACT	ADDRESS/ NOTE
SESSION 10				
SESSION 11				
SESSION 12				
SESSION 13				
SESSION 14				
SESSION 15				
SESSION 16				
SESSION 17				
SESSION 18				
SESSION 19				
SESSION 20				

	DATE/TIME	THERAPIST	THERAPIST CONTACT	ADDRESS/ NOTE
SESSION 21				
SESSION 22				
SESSION 23				
SESSION 24				
SESSION 25				
SESSION 26				
SESSION 27				
SESSION 28				
SESSION 29				
SESSION 30				

Therapy Goals

Write your goal(s) for your therapy sessions and the actions you need to take to achieve them. (Come back and review your goals whenever is necessary. Eg: Every 3 months)

Example

GOAL & ACTIONS: *Overcoming depression after a break up*   **DATE:**

I will start exercising again – 3 times a week at least, for 45 minutes each time

I will stop refusing my firends invitations to get together; I will socialize again

I will journal briefly every day, answering this: what are you proud of having done today?

GOAL & ACTIONS: **DATE:**

ACTIONS:

_____

_____

_____

GOAL & ACTIONS: **DATE:**

ACTIONS:

_____

_____

_____

GOAL & ACTIONS: **DATE:**

ACTIONS:

_____

_____

_____

Therapy Tools I Learned

Therapy tools can help you throughout your journey. Whenever you learn about a helpful tool capture it here so that you can easily refer back to it when you need it.

TOOL: *Journaling*

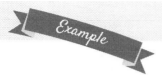

DESCRIPTION / RELEVANT NOTES:

My therapist suggested that I write down the things that make me happy during the day. And also to write down when I feel confused and unable to make a decision.

I love this "journaling tool" because I fell more relaxed and less anxious as I vent my thoughts. It also helps me to feel more focused and organized because I gain more clarity on how to prioritize what is really important to me.

TOOL: **DATE:**

DESCRIPTION / RELEVANT NOTES:

TOOL: **DATE:**

DESCRIPTION / RELEVANT NOTES:

TOOL: **DATE:**

DESCRIPTION / RELEVANT NOTES:

Therapy Tools I Learned

TOOL: DATE:

DESCRIPTION / RELEVANT NOTES:

TOOL: DATE:

DESCRIPTION / RELEVANT NOTES:

TOOL: DATE:

DESCRIPTION / RELEVANT NOTES:

TOOL: DATE:

DESCRIPTION / RELEVANT NOTES:

Therapy Session Notes

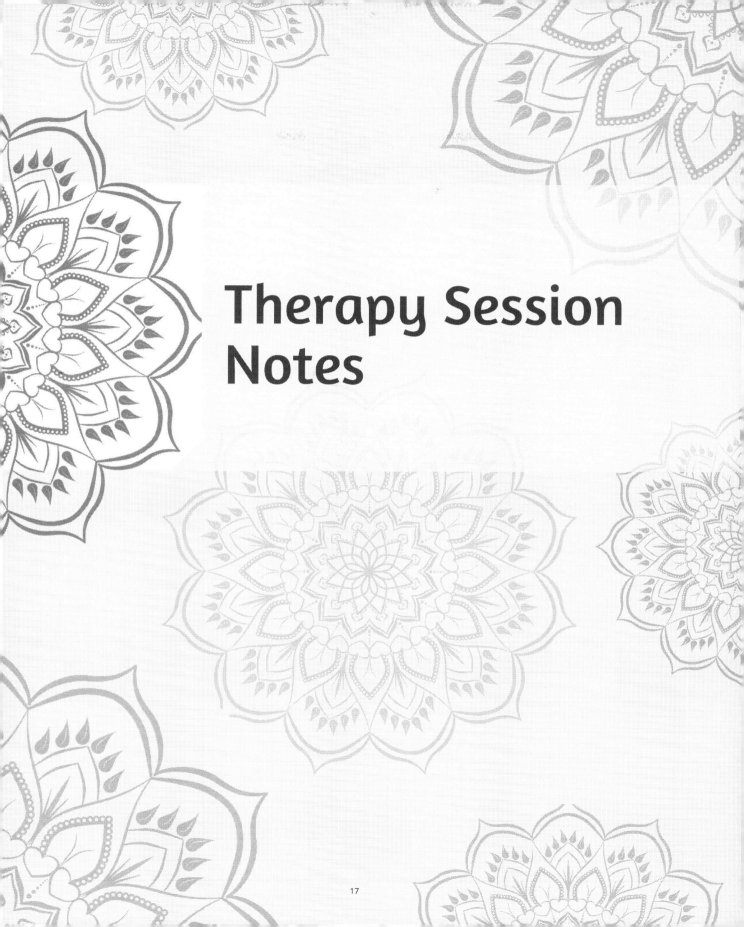

Session Date:

Session #:

Next Session Date:

Pre and Post Session Tracker:

Before the Session:

My Mood is: ☹ 😟(crossed out) 😐 🙂 😀

How do I feel physically?
(In a scale 1 - 5, with 5 being the best)
☐ ☐ ☐ ☑ ☐

How do I feel emotionally?
(In a scale 1 - 5, with 5 being the best)
☐ ☑ ☐ ☐ ☐

How is the quality of my sleep?
(In a scale 1 - 5, with 5 being the best)
☐ ☑ ☐ ☐ ☐

How was my week in general?
(In a scale 1 - 5, with 5 being the best)
☐ ☐ ☑ ☐ ☐

After the Session:

My Mood is: ☹ ☹ 😐 🙂(crossed out) 😀

Did I feel heard & comfortable?
(In a scale 1 - 5, with 5 being the best)
☐ ☐ ☐ ☐ ☑

How do I feel emotionally now?
(In a scale 1 - 5, with 5 being the best)
☐ ☐ ☐ ☑ ☐

Did this session give me ideas / clarify my thoughts about what to do next?
(In a scale 1 - 5, with 5 being the best)
☐ ☐ ☐ ☐ ☑

How helpful this session was?
(In a scale 1 - 5, with 5 being the best)
☐ ☐ ☐ ☐ ☑

Topic(s) I want to discuss and/or goal(s) my therapist suggested for the session:

(+Optional Reflection ideas: How do I feel about these things / how do they affect my life? Do I already see ways to help myself to get over them?)

My partner is acting in a strange way, which makes me feel very uncomfortable. It feels as if we need to have an important conversation, but none of us takes the first step. Is it fear?

If this is the end of our relationship, I really don't know what I should do. I would feel embarrassed to be separated once again. Plus, financially it would be a struggle to be on my own.

And because of the pandemic, I haven't opened up or had fun times with others in a long time. So I feel very lonely, although technically we are at home together every night.

This confusion paralyzes me. I want to understand if it is better to talk to him and face the consequences, or keep this situation going at least during the pandemic...

I have been reading Instagram posts about how to have a healthy relationship, but I know that this is not enough, especially if I don't take any acion with the new information that I read.

Notes from Session: relevant comments & insights.

Reminder: Write here possible actions / "homework" suggested by the therapist

(Complete during or after the session)

My therapist suggested some things really interesting that I can apply while having the conversation with my partner (and in other situations, too).

- Be open about your discomfort:

She said that I could say: "Look, Richard, I really don't know how to have this conversation, this is hard for me too, so I apologize in advance if it doesn't sound so smooth. But I want to tell you about how I've been feeling..."

- As much as possible, talk about you/your feelings, not the other

She suggested that instead of complaining about his behavior, I talk about how I feel. For instance, instead of saying how much I hate when he spends all evening on the computer instead of talking to me, I could say: "I've been feeling really lonely, I miss doing things together with you..."

- She reminded me to give ideas of what to do next

"What if we start watching a Netflix show together? Or take that programming class online, which could help us both in our careers? And maybe we can start having dinners outside once a week, too, since the vaccination rates are high in our neighborhood and we have the option of eating outdoors."

- Finally, she reminded me that if the relationship is over, I will be able to move on with my life

I overcame much more difficult situations in the past. While breaking up would be painful, I can probably recover from it. And I could live with my sister for a few months, avoiding the need to pay rent on my own...

The main things that I want to remember from today are:

(Some ideas: Homework, key takeaways, reminders for your next session, challenges to keep in mind and wins to be celebrated!)

■ After talking to my therapist today, I decided to have the conversation with Richard

■ This conversation will not be easy, but avoiding it is making me miserable already. Having the conversation will probably help things change, hopefully for the better

■ Even though I lost my job, I'm a capable woman and I'll be able to find a way back to the workplace and become independent again

Session Date:

Session #:

Next Session Date:

Pre and Post Session Tracker:

Before the Session:	After the Session:

My Mood is: ☹ ☹ 😐 ☺ 😃

How do I feel physically?
(In a scale 1 - 5, with 5 being the best)
☐☐☐☐☐

How do I feel emotionally?
(In a scale 1 - 5, with 5 being the best)
☐☐☐☐☐

How is the quality of my sleep?
(In a scale 1 - 5, with 5 being the best)
☐☐☐☐☐

How was my week in general?
(In a scale 1 - 5, with 5 being the best)
☐☐☐☐☐

My Mood is: ☹ ☹ 😐 ☺ 😃

Did I feel heard & comfortable?
(In a scale 1 - 5, with 5 being the best)
☐☐☐☐☐

How do I feel emotionally now?
(In a scale 1 - 5, with 5 being the best)
☐☐☐☐☐

Did this session give me ideas / clarify my thoughts about what to do next?
(In a scale 1 - 5, with 5 being the best)
☐☐☐☐☐

How helpful this session was?
(In a scale 1 - 5, with 5 being the best)
☐☐☐☐☐

Topic(s) I want to discuss and/or goal(s) my therapist suggested for the session:

(+Optional Reflection ideas: How do I feel about these things / how do they affect my life? Do I already see ways to help myself to get over them?)

Notes from Session: relevant comments & insights.

Reminder: Write here possible actions / "homework" suggested by the therapist

(Complete during or after the session)

The main things that I want to remember from today are:

(Some ideas: Homework, key takeaways, reminders for your next session, challenges to keep in mind and wins to be celebrated!)

- ■
- ■
- ■

Session Date:

Next Session Date:

Session #:

Pre and Post Session Tracker:

<u>Before the Session:</u>

My Mood is: ☹ ☹ ☺ ☺ ☺

How do I feel physically?
(In a scale 1 - 5, with 5 being the best)
☐☐☐☐☐

How do I feel emotionally?
(In a scale 1 - 5, with 5 being the best)
☐☐☐☐☐

How is the quality of my sleep?
(In a scale 1 - 5, with 5 being the best)
☐☐☐☐☐

How was my week in general?
(In a scale 1 - 5, with 5 being the best)
☐☐☐☐☐

<u>After the Session:</u>

My Mood is: ☹ ☹ ☺ ☺ ☺

Did I feel heard & comfortable?
(In a scale 1 - 5, with 5 being the best)
☐☐☐☐☐

How do I feel emotionally now?
(In a scale 1 - 5, with 5 being the best)
☐☐☐☐☐

Did this session give me ideas / clarify my thoughts about what to do next?
(In a scale 1 - 5, with 5 being the best)
☐☐☐☐☐

How helpful this session was?
(In a scale 1 - 5, with 5 being the best)
☐☐☐☐☐

Topic(s) I want to discuss and/or goal(s) my therapist suggested for the session:

(+Optional Reflection ideas: How do I feel about these things / how do they affect my life? Do I already see ways to help myself to get over them?)

Notes from Session: relevant comments & insights.

Reminder: Write here possible actions / "homework" suggested by the therapist

(Complete during or after the session)

The main things that I want to remember from today are:

(Some ideas: Homework, key takeaways, reminders for your next session, challenges to keep in mind and wins to be celebrated!)

- ☐
- ☐
- ☐

Session Date:

Session #:

Next Session Date:

Pre and Post Session Tracker:

Before the Session:

My Mood is: ☹ 🙁 😐 🙂 😄

How do I feel physically?
(In a scale 1 - 5, with 5 being the best)
☐ ☐ ☐ ☐ ☐

How do I feel emotionally?
(In a scale 1 - 5, with 5 being the best)
☐ ☐ ☐ ☐ ☐

How is the quality of my sleep?
(In a scale 1 - 5, with 5 being the best)
☐ ☐ ☐ ☐ ☐

How was my week in general?
(In a scale 1 - 5, with 5 being the best)
☐ ☐ ☐ ☐ ☐

After the Session:

My Mood is: ☹ 🙁 😐 🙂 😄

Did I feel heard & comfortable?
(In a scale 1 - 5, with 5 being the best)
☐ ☐ ☐ ☐ ☐

How do I feel emotionally now?
(In a scale 1 - 5, with 5 being the best)
☐ ☐ ☐ ☐ ☐

Did this session give me ideas / clarify my thoughts about what to do next?
(In a scale 1 - 5, with 5 being the best)
☐ ☐ ☐ ☐ ☐

How helpful this session was?
(In a scale 1 - 5, with 5 being the best)
☐ ☐ ☐ ☐ ☐

Topic(s) I want to discuss and/or goal(s) my therapist suggested for the session:

(+Optional Reflection ideas: How do I feel about these things / how do they affect my life? Do I already see ways to help myself to get over them?)

Notes from Session: relevant comments & insights.

Reminder: Write here possible actions / "homework" suggested by the therapist

(Complete during or after the session)

The main things that I want to remember from today are:

(Some ideas: Homework, key takeaways, reminders for your next session,
challenges to keep in mind and wins to be celebrated!)

- ■
- ■
- ■

Session Date:

Session #:

Next Session Date:

Pre and Post Session Tracker:

Before the Session:		After the Session:	
My Mood is: ☹ ☹ 😐 🙂 😀		**My Mood is:** ☹ ☹ 😐 🙂 😀	
How do I feel physically? (In a scale 1 – 5, with 5 being the best)	☐☐☐☐☐	**Did I feel heard & comfortable?** (In a scale 1 – 5, with 5 being the best)	☐☐☐☐☐
How do I feel emotionally? (In a scale 1 – 5, with 5 being the best)	☐☐☐☐☐	**How do I feel emotionally now?** (In a scale 1 – 5, with 5 being the best)	☐☐☐☐☐
How is the quality of my sleep? (In a scale 1 – 5, with 5 being the best)	☐☐☐☐☐	**Did this session give me ideas / clarify my thoughts about what to do next?** (In a scale 1 – 5, with 5 being the best)	☐☐☐☐☐
How was my week in general? (In a scale 1 – 5, with 5 being the best)	☐☐☐☐☐	**How helpful this session was?** (In a scale 1 – 5, with 5 being the best)	☐☐☐☐☐

Topic(s) I want to discuss and/or goal(s) my therapist suggested for the session:

(+Optional Reflection ideas: How do I feel about these things / how do they affect my life? Do I already see ways to help myself to get over them?)

Notes from Session: relevant comments & insights.

Reminder: Write here possible actions / "homework" suggested by the therapist

(Complete during or after the session)

The main things that I want to remember from today are:

(Some ideas: Homework, key takeaways, reminders for your next session, challenges to keep in mind and wins to be celebrated!)

■

■

■

Session Date:

Session #:

Next Session Date:

Pre and Post Session Tracker:

Before the Session:

My Mood is: ☹ ☹ 😐 🙂 😃

How do I feel physically?
(In a scale 1 - 5, with 5 being the best)
☐ ☐ ☐ ☐ ☐

How do I feel emotionally?
(In a scale 1 - 5, with 5 being the best)
☐ ☐ ☐ ☐ ☐

How is the quality of my sleep?
(In a scale 1 - 5, with 5 being the best)
☐ ☐ ☐ ☐ ☐

How was my week in general?
(In a scale 1 - 5, with 5 being the best)
☐ ☐ ☐ ☐ ☐

After the Session:

My Mood is: ☹ ☹ 😐 🙂 😃

Did I feel heard & comfortable?
(In a scale 1 - 5, with 5 being the best)
☐ ☐ ☐ ☐ ☐

How do I feel emotionally now?
(In a scale 1 - 5, with 5 being the best)
☐ ☐ ☐ ☐ ☐

Did this session give me ideas / clarify my thoughts about what to do next?
(In a scale 1 - 5, with 5 being the best)
☐ ☐ ☐ ☐ ☐

How helpful this session was?
(In a scale 1 - 5, with 5 being the best)
☐ ☐ ☐ ☐ ☐

Topic(s) I want to discuss and/or goal(s) my therapist suggested for the session:

(+Optional Reflection ideas: How do I feel about these things / how do they affect my life? Do I already see ways to help myself to get over them?)

Notes from Session: relevant comments & insights.

Reminder: Write here possible actions / "homework" suggested by the therapist

(Complete during or after the session)

The main things that I want to remember from today are:

(Some ideas: Homework, key takeaways, reminders for your next session,
challenges to keep in mind and wins to be celebrated!)

- ■
- ■
- ■

Session Date:

Next Session Date:

Session #:

Pre and Post Session Tracker:

Before the Session:

My Mood is: ☹ ☹ 😐 🙂 😃

How do I feel physically?
(In a scale 1 - 5, with 5 being the best)
☐ ☐ ☐ ☐ ☐

How do I feel emotionally?
(In a scale 1 - 5, with 5 being the best)
☐ ☐ ☐ ☐ ☐

How is the quality of my sleep?
(In a scale 1 - 5, with 5 being the best)
☐ ☐ ☐ ☐ ☐

How was my week in general?
(In a scale 1 - 5, with 5 being the best)
☐ ☐ ☐ ☐ ☐

After the Session:

My Mood is: ☹ ☹ 😐 🙂 😃

Did I feel heard & comfortable?
(In a scale 1 - 5, with 5 being the best)
☐ ☐ ☐ ☐ ☐

How do I feel emotionally now?
(In a scale 1 - 5, with 5 being the best)
☐ ☐ ☐ ☐ ☐

Did this session give me ideas / clarify my thoughts about what to do next?
(In a scale 1 - 5, with 5 being the best)
☐ ☐ ☐ ☐ ☐

How helpful this session was?
(In a scale 1 - 5, with 5 being the best)
☐ ☐ ☐ ☐ ☐

Topic(s) I want to discuss and/or goal(s) my therapist suggested for the session:

(+Optional Reflection ideas: How do I feel about these things / how do they affect my life? Do I already see ways to help myself to get over them?)

Notes from Session: relevant comments & insights.

Reminder: Write here possible actions / "homework" suggested by the therapist

(Complete during or after the session)

The main things that I want to remember from today are:

(Some ideas: Homework, key takeaways, reminders for your next session,
challenges to keep in mind and wins to be celebrated!)

- ■
- ■
- ■

Session Date:

Session #:

Next Session Date:

Pre and Post Session Tracker:

Before the Session:

My Mood is: 😟 😕 😐 🙂 😃

How do I feel physically?
(In a scale 1 - 5, with 5 being the best)
☐ ☐ ☐ ☐ ☐

How do I feel emotionally?
(In a scale 1 - 5, with 5 being the best)
☐ ☐ ☐ ☐ ☐

How is the quality of my sleep?
(In a scale 1 - 5, with 5 being the best)
☐ ☐ ☐ ☐ ☐

How was my week in general?
(In a scale 1 - 5, with 5 being the best)
☐ ☐ ☐ ☐ ☐

After the Session:

My Mood is: 😟 😕 😐 🙂 😃

Did I feel heard & comfortable?
(In a scale 1 - 5, with 5 being the best)
☐ ☐ ☐ ☐ ☐

How do I feel emotionally now?
(In a scale 1 - 5, with 5 being the best)
☐ ☐ ☐ ☐ ☐

Did this session give me ideas / clarify my thoughts about what to do next?
(In a scale 1 - 5, with 5 being the best)
☐ ☐ ☐ ☐ ☐

How helpful this session was?
(In a scale 1 - 5, with 5 being the best)
☐ ☐ ☐ ☐ ☐

Topic(s) I want to discuss and/or goal(s) my therapist suggested for the session:

(+Optional Reflection ideas: How do I feel about these things / how do they affect my life? Do I already see ways to help myself to get over them?)

Notes from Session: relevant comments & insights.

Reminder: Write here possible actions / "homework" suggested by the therapist

(Complete during or after the session)

The main things that I want to remember from today are:

(Some ideas: Homework, key takeaways, reminders for your next session,
challenges to keep in mind and wins to be celebrated!)

- ■
- ■
- ■

Session Date:

Session #:

Next Session Date:

Pre and Post Session Tracker:

Before the Session:

My Mood is: ☹ ☹ 😐 🙂 😃

How do I feel physically?
(In a scale 1 - 5, with 5 being the best)
☐ ☐ ☐ ☐ ☐

How do I feel emotionally?
(In a scale 1 - 5, with 5 being the best)
☐ ☐ ☐ ☐ ☐

How is the quality of my sleep?
(In a scale 1 - 5, with 5 being the best)
☐ ☐ ☐ ☐ ☐

How was my week in general?
(In a scale 1 - 5, with 5 being the best)
☐ ☐ ☐ ☐ ☐

After the Session:

My Mood is: ☹ ☹ 😐 🙂 😃

Did I feel heard & comfortable?
(In a scale 1 - 5, with 5 being the best)
☐ ☐ ☐ ☐ ☐

How do I feel emotionally now?
(In a scale 1 - 5, with 5 being the best)
☐ ☐ ☐ ☐ ☐

**Did this session give me ideas /
clarify my thoughts about what to
do next?**
(In a scale 1 - 5, with 5 being the best)
☐ ☐ ☐ ☐ ☐

How helpful this session was?
(In a scale 1 - 5, with 5 being the best)
☐ ☐ ☐ ☐ ☐

Topic(s) I want to discuss and/or goal(s) my therapist suggested for the session:

(+Optional Reflection ideas: How do I feel about these things / how do they affect my life?
Do I already see ways to help myself to get over them?)

Notes from Session: relevant comments & insights.

Reminder: Write here possible actions / "homework" suggested by the therapist

(Complete during or after the session)

The main things that I want to remember from today are:

(Some ideas: Homework, key takeaways, reminders for your next session,
challenges to keep in mind and wins to be celebrated!)

- ▪
- ▪
- ▪

Session Date:

Session #:

Next Session Date:

Pre and Post Session Tracker:

Before the Session:		After the Session:	
My Mood is: ☹ ☹ 😐 ☺ 😄		**My Mood is:** ☹ ☹ 😐 ☺ 😄	
How do I feel physically? (In a scale 1 - 5, with 5 being the best)	☐☐☐☐☐	**Did I feel heard & comfortable?** (In a scale 1 - 5, with 5 being the best)	☐☐☐☐☐
How do I feel emotionally? (In a scale 1 - 5, with 5 being the best)	☐☐☐☐☐	**How do I feel emotionally now?** (In a scale 1 - 5, with 5 being the best)	☐☐☐☐☐
How is the quality of my sleep? (In a scale 1 - 5, with 5 being the best)	☐☐☐☐☐	**Did this session give me ideas / clarify my thoughts about what to do next?** (In a scale 1 - 5, with 5 being the best)	☐☐☐☐☐
How was my week in general? (In a scale 1 - 5, with 5 being the best)	☐☐☐☐☐	**How helpful this session was?** (In a scale 1 - 5, with 5 being the best)	☐☐☐☐☐

Topic(s) I want to discuss and/or goal(s) my therapist suggested for the session:

(+Optional Reflection ideas: How do I feel about these things / how do they affect my life? Do I already see ways to help myself to get over them?)

Notes from Session: relevant comments & insights.

Reminder: Write here possible actions / "homework" suggested by the therapist

(Complete during or after the session)

The main things that I want to remember from today are:

(Some ideas: Homework, key takeaways, reminders for your next session,
challenges to keep in mind and wins to be celebrated!)

- ▪
- ▪
- ▪

Session Date:

Session #:

Next Session Date:

Pre and Post Session Tracker:

Before the Session:	After the Session:
My Mood is: 😟 😦 😐 🙂 😀	**My Mood is:** 😟 😦 😐 🙂 😀
How do I feel physically? (In a scale 1 - 5, with 5 being the best) ☐☐☐☐☐	**Did I feel heard & comfortable?** (In a scale 1 - 5, with 5 being the best) ☐☐☐☐☐
How do I feel emotionally? (In a scale 1 - 5, with 5 being the best) ☐☐☐☐☐	**How do I feel emotionally now?** (In a scale 1 - 5, with 5 being the best) ☐☐☐☐☐
How is the quality of my sleep? (In a scale 1 - 5, with 5 being the best) ☐☐☐☐☐	**Did this session give me ideas / clarify my thoughts about what to do next?** (In a scale 1 - 5, with 5 being the best) ☐☐☐☐☐
How was my week in general? (In a scale 1 - 5, with 5 being the best) ☐☐☐☐☐	**How helpful this session was?** (In a scale 1 - 5, with 5 being the best) ☐☐☐☐☐

Topic(s) I want to discuss and/or goal(s) my therapist suggested for the session:

(+Optional Reflection ideas: How do I feel about these things / how do they affect my life? Do I already see ways to help myself to get over them?)

Notes from Session: relevant comments & insights.

Reminder: Write here possible actions / "homework" suggested by the therapist

(Complete during or after the session)

The main things that I want to remember from today are:

(Some ideas: Homework, key takeaways, reminders for your next session, challenges to keep in mind and wins to be celebrated!)

- ▪
- ▪
- ▪

Session Date:

Session #:

Next Session Date:

Pre and Post Session Tracker:

Before the Session:

My Mood is: ☹ 🙁 😐 🙂 😃

How do I feel physically?
(In a scale 1 - 5, with 5 being the best) ☐ ☐ ☐ ☐ ☐

How do I feel emotionally?
(In a scale 1 - 5, with 5 being the best) ☐ ☐ ☐ ☐ ☐

How is the quality of my sleep?
(In a scale 1 - 5, with 5 being the best) ☐ ☐ ☐ ☐ ☐

How was my week in general?
(In a scale 1 - 5, with 5 being the best) ☐ ☐ ☐ ☐ ☐

After the Session:

My Mood is: ☹ 🙁 😐 🙂 😃

Did I feel heard & comfortable?
(In a scale 1 - 5, with 5 being the best) ☐ ☐ ☐ ☐ ☐

How do I feel emotionally now?
(In a scale 1 - 5, with 5 being the best) ☐ ☐ ☐ ☐ ☐

**Did this session give me ideas /
clarify my thoughts about what to
do next?**
(In a scale 1 - 5, with 5 being the best) ☐ ☐ ☐ ☐ ☐

How helpful this session was?
(In a scale 1 - 5, with 5 being the best) ☐ ☐ ☐ ☐ ☐

Topic(s) I want to discuss and/or goal(s) my therapist suggested for the session:

(+Optional Reflection ideas: How do I feel about these things / how do they affect my life?
Do I already see ways to help myself to get over them?)

Notes from Session: relevant comments & insights.

Reminder: Write here possible actions / "homework" suggested by the therapist

(Complete during or after the session)

The main things that I want to remember from today are:

(Some ideas: Homework, key takeaways, reminders for your next session,
challenges to keep in mind and wins to be celebrated!)

- ▪
- ▪
- ▪

Session Date:

Session #:

Next Session Date:

Pre and Post Session Tracker:

Before the Session:

My Mood is: 😞 😟 😐 🙂 😀

How do I feel physically?
(In a scale 1 - 5, with 5 being the best)
☐ ☐ ☐ ☐ ☐

How do I feel emotionally?
(In a scale 1 - 5, with 5 being the best)
☐ ☐ ☐ ☐ ☐

How is the quality of my sleep?
(In a scale 1 - 5, with 5 being the best)
☐ ☐ ☐ ☐ ☐

How was my week in general?
(In a scale 1 - 5, with 5 being the best)
☐ ☐ ☐ ☐ ☐

After the Session:

My Mood is: 😞 😟 😐 🙂 😀

Did I feel heard & comfortable?
(In a scale 1 - 5, with 5 being the best)
☐ ☐ ☐ ☐ ☐

How do I feel emotionally now?
(In a scale 1 - 5, with 5 being the best)
☐ ☐ ☐ ☐ ☐

Did this session give me ideas / clarify my thoughts about what to do next?
(In a scale 1 - 5, with 5 being the best)
☐ ☐ ☐ ☐ ☐

How helpful this session was?
(In a scale 1 - 5, with 5 being the best)
☐ ☐ ☐ ☐ ☐

Topic(s) I want to discuss and/or goal(s) my therapist suggested for the session:

(+Optional Reflection ideas: How do I feel about these things / how do they affect my life? Do I already see ways to help myself to get over them?)

Notes from Session: relevant comments & insights.

Reminder: Write here possible actions / "homework" suggested by the therapist

(Complete during or after the session)

The main things that I want to remember from today are:

(Some ideas: Homework, key takeaways, reminders for your next session,
challenges to keep in mind and wins to be celebrated!)

- ◼
- ◼
- ◼

Session Date:

Session #:

Next Session Date:

Pre and Post Session Tracker:

Before the Session:

My Mood is: ☹ 🙁 😐 🙂 😄

How do I feel physically?
(In a scale 1 - 5, with 5 being the best)
☐ ☐ ☐ ☐ ☐

How do I feel emotionally?
(In a scale 1 - 5, with 5 being the best)
☐ ☐ ☐ ☐ ☐

How is the quality of my sleep?
(In a scale 1 - 5, with 5 being the best)
☐ ☐ ☐ ☐ ☐

How was my week in general?
(In a scale 1 - 5, with 5 being the best)
☐ ☐ ☐ ☐ ☐

After the Session:

My Mood is: ☹ 🙁 😐 🙂 😄

Did I feel heard & comfortable?
(In a scale 1 - 5, with 5 being the best)
☐ ☐ ☐ ☐ ☐

How do I feel emotionally now?
(In a scale 1 - 5, with 5 being the best)
☐ ☐ ☐ ☐ ☐

**Did this session give me ideas /
clarify my thoughts about what to
do next?**
(In a scale 1 - 5, with 5 being the best)
☐ ☐ ☐ ☐ ☐

How helpful this session was?
(In a scale 1 - 5, with 5 being the best)
☐ ☐ ☐ ☐ ☐

Topic(s) I want to discuss and/or goal(s) my therapist suggested for the session:

(+Optional Reflection ideas: How do I feel about these things / how do they affect my life?
Do I already see ways to help myself to get over them?)

Notes from Session: relevant comments & insights.

Reminder: Write here possible actions / "homework" suggested by the therapist

(Complete during or after the session)

The main things that I want to remember from today are:

(Some ideas: Homework, key takeaways, reminders for your next session,
challenges to keep in mind and wins to be celebrated!)

-
-
-

Session Date:

Session #:

Next Session Date:

Pre and Post Session Tracker:

Before the Session:	After the Session:

My Mood is: 😟 😕 😐 🙂 😄   **My Mood is:** 😟 😕 😐 🙂 😄

How do I feel physically?
(In a scale 1 - 5, with 5 being the best)   ☐☐☐☐☐

Did I feel heard & comfortable?
(In a scale 1 - 5, with 5 being the best)   ☐☐☐☐☐

How do I feel emotionally?
(In a scale 1 - 5, with 5 being the best)   ☐☐☐☐☐

How do I feel emotionally now?
(In a scale 1 - 5, with 5 being the best)   ☐☐☐☐☐

How is the quality of my sleep?
(In a scale 1 - 5, with 5 being the best)   ☐☐☐☐☐

**Did this session give me ideas /
clarify my thoughts about what to
do next?**
(In a scale 1 - 5, with 5 being the best)   ☐☐☐☐☐

How was my week in general?
(In a scale 1 - 5, with 5 being the best)   ☐☐☐☐☐

How helpful this session was?
(In a scale 1 - 5, with 5 being the best)   ☐☐☐☐☐

Topic(s) I want to discuss and/or goal(s) my therapist suggested for the session:

(+Optional Reflection ideas: How do I feel about these things / how do they affect my life?
Do I already see ways to help myself to get over them?)

Notes from Session: relevant comments & insights.

Reminder: Write here possible actions / "homework" suggested by the therapist

(Complete during or after the session)

The main things that I want to remember from today are:

(Some ideas: Homework, key takeaways, reminders for your next session, challenges to keep in mind and wins to be celebrated!)

- ■
- ■
- ■

Session Date:

Session #:

Next Session Date:

Pre and Post Session Tracker:

Before the Session:

My Mood is: 😟 😕 😐 🙂 😃

How do I feel physically?
(In a scale 1 - 5, with 5 being the best)
☐ ☐ ☐ ☐ ☐

How do I feel emotionally?
(In a scale 1 - 5, with 5 being the best)
☐ ☐ ☐ ☐ ☐

How is the quality of my sleep?
(In a scale 1 - 5, with 5 being the best)
☐ ☐ ☐ ☐ ☐

How was my week in general?
(In a scale 1 - 5, with 5 being the best)
☐ ☐ ☐ ☐ ☐

After the Session:

My Mood is: 😟 😕 😐 🙂 😃

Did I feel heard & comfortable?
(In a scale 1 - 5, with 5 being the best)
☐ ☐ ☐ ☐ ☐

How do I feel emotionally now?
(In a scale 1 - 5, with 5 being the best)
☐ ☐ ☐ ☐ ☐

Did this session give me ideas / clarify my thoughts about what to do next?
(In a scale 1 - 5, with 5 being the best)
☐ ☐ ☐ ☐ ☐

How helpful this session was?
(In a scale 1 - 5, with 5 being the best)
☐ ☐ ☐ ☐ ☐

Topic(s) I want to discuss and/or goal(s) my therapist suggested for the session:

(+Optional Reflection ideas: How do I feel about these things / how do they affect my life? Do I already see ways to help myself to get over them?)

Notes from Session: relevant comments & insights.

Reminder: Write here possible actions / "homework" suggested by the therapist

(Complete during or after the session)

The main things that I want to remember from today are:

(Some ideas: Homework, key takeaways, reminders for your next session,
challenges to keep in mind and wins to be celebrated!)

- ■
- ■
- ■

Session Date:

Session #:

Next Session Date:

Pre and Post Session Tracker:

Before the Session:

My Mood is: ☹ 🙁 😐 🙂 😄

How do I feel physically?
(In a scale 1 - 5, with 5 being the best)
☐ ☐ ☐ ☐ ☐

How do I feel emotionally?
(In a scale 1 - 5, with 5 being the best)
☐ ☐ ☐ ☐ ☐

How is the quality of my sleep?
(In a scale 1 - 5, with 5 being the best)
☐ ☐ ☐ ☐ ☐

How was my week in general?
(In a scale 1 - 5, with 5 being the best)
☐ ☐ ☐ ☐ ☐

After the Session:

My Mood is: ☹ 🙁 😐 🙂 😄

Did I feel heard & comfortable?
(In a scale 1 - 5, with 5 being the best)
☐ ☐ ☐ ☐ ☐

How do I feel emotionally now?
(In a scale 1 - 5, with 5 being the best)
☐ ☐ ☐ ☐ ☐

**Did this session give me ideas /
clarify my thoughts about what to
do next?**
(In a scale 1 - 5, with 5 being the best)
☐ ☐ ☐ ☐ ☐

How helpful this session was?
(In a scale 1 - 5, with 5 being the best)
☐ ☐ ☐ ☐ ☐

Topic(s) I want to discuss and/or goal(s) my therapist suggested for the session:

(+Optional Reflection ideas: How do I feel about these things / how do they affect my life?
Do I already see ways to help myself to get over them?)

Notes from Session: relevant comments & insights.

Reminder: Write here possible actions / "homework" suggested by the therapist

(Complete during or after the session)

The main things that I want to remember from today are:

(Some ideas: Homework, key takeaways, reminders for your next session, challenges to keep in mind and wins to be celebrated!)

- ◼
- ◼
- ◼

Session Date:

Session #:

Next Session Date:

Pre and Post Session Tracker:

Before the Session:	After the Session:

My Mood is: ☹ ☹ 😐 🙂 😀

How do I feel physically?
(In a scale 1 - 5, with 5 being the best)
☐ ☐ ☐ ☐ ☐

How do I feel emotionally?
(In a scale 1 - 5, with 5 being the best)
☐ ☐ ☐ ☐ ☐

How is the quality of my sleep?
(In a scale 1 - 5, with 5 being the best)
☐ ☐ ☐ ☐ ☐

How was my week in general?
(In a scale 1 - 5, with 5 being the best)
☐ ☐ ☐ ☐ ☐

My Mood is: ☹ ☹ 😐 🙂 😀

Did I feel heard & comfortable?
(In a scale 1 - 5, with 5 being the best)
☐ ☐ ☐ ☐ ☐

How do I feel emotionally now?
(In a scale 1 - 5, with 5 being the best)
☐ ☐ ☐ ☐ ☐

Did this session give me ideas / clarify my thoughts about what to do next?
(In a scale 1 - 5, with 5 being the best)
☐ ☐ ☐ ☐ ☐

How helpful this session was?
(In a scale 1 - 5, with 5 being the best)
☐ ☐ ☐ ☐ ☐

Topic(s) I want to discuss and/or goal(s) my therapist suggested for the session:

(+Optional Reflection ideas: How do I feel about these things / how do they affect my life? Do I already see ways to help myself to get over them?)

Notes from Session: relevant comments & insights.

Reminder: Write here possible actions / "homework" suggested by the therapist

(Complete during or after the session)

The main things that I want to remember from today are:

(Some ideas: Homework, key takeaways, reminders for your next session, challenges to keep in mind and wins to be celebrated!)

■

■

■

Session Date:

Session #:

Next Session Date:

Pre and Post Session Tracker:

Before the Session:

My Mood is: ☹ ☹ 😐 ☺ 😀

How do I feel physically?
(In a scale 1 - 5, with 5 being the best)
☐ ☐ ☐ ☐ ☐

How do I feel emotionally?
(In a scale 1 - 5, with 5 being the best)
☐ ☐ ☐ ☐ ☐

How is the quality of my sleep?
(In a scale 1 - 5, with 5 being the best)
☐ ☐ ☐ ☐ ☐

How was my week in general?
(In a scale 1 - 5, with 5 being the best)
☐ ☐ ☐ ☐ ☐

After the Session:

My Mood is: ☹ ☹ 😐 ☺ 😀

Did I feel heard & comfortable?
(In a scale 1 - 5, with 5 being the best)
☐ ☐ ☐ ☐ ☐

How do I feel emotionally now?
(In a scale 1 - 5, with 5 being the best)
☐ ☐ ☐ ☐ ☐

**Did this session give me ideas /
clarify my thoughts about what to
do next?**
(In a scale 1 - 5, with 5 being the best)
☐ ☐ ☐ ☐ ☐

How helpful this session was?
(In a scale 1 - 5, with 5 being the best)
☐ ☐ ☐ ☐ ☐

Topic(s) I want to discuss and/or goal(s) my therapist suggested for the session:

(+Optional Reflection ideas: How do I feel about these things / how do they affect my life?
Do I already see ways to help myself to get over them?)

Notes from Session: relevant comments & insights.

Reminder: Write here possible actions / "homework" suggested by the therapist

(Complete during or after the session)

The main things that I want to remember from today are:

(Some ideas: Homework, key takeaways, reminders for your next session,
challenges to keep in mind and wins to be celebrated!)

- ◼
- ◼
- ◼

Session Date:

Session #:

Next Session Date:

Pre and Post Session Tracker:

Before the Session:

My Mood is: ☹ ☹ 😐 🙂 😄

How do I feel physically?
(In a scale 1 - 5, with 5 being the best)
☐ ☐ ☐ ☐ ☐

How do I feel emotionally?
(In a scale 1 - 5, with 5 being the best)
☐ ☐ ☐ ☐ ☐

How is the quality of my sleep?
(In a scale 1 - 5, with 5 being the best)
☐ ☐ ☐ ☐ ☐

How was my week in general?
(In a scale 1 - 5, with 5 being the best)
☐ ☐ ☐ ☐ ☐

After the Session:

My Mood is: ☹ ☹ 😐 🙂 😄

Did I feel heard & comfortable?
(In a scale 1 - 5, with 5 being the best)
☐ ☐ ☐ ☐ ☐

How do I feel emotionally now?
(In a scale 1 - 5, with 5 being the best)
☐ ☐ ☐ ☐ ☐

Did this session give me ideas / clarify my thoughts about what to do next?
(In a scale 1 - 5, with 5 being the best)
☐ ☐ ☐ ☐ ☐

How helpful this session was?
(In a scale 1 - 5, with 5 being the best)
☐ ☐ ☐ ☐ ☐

Topic(s) I want to discuss and/or goal(s) my therapist suggested for the session:

(+Optional Reflection ideas: How do I feel about these things / how do they affect my life? Do I already see ways to help myself to get over them?)

Notes from Session: relevant comments & insights.

Reminder: Write here possible actions / "homework" suggested by the therapist

(Complete during or after the session)

The main things that I want to remember from today are:

(Some ideas: Homework, key takeaways, reminders for your next session, challenges to keep in mind and wins to be celebrated!)

- ■
- ■
- ■

Session Date:

Session #:

Next Session Date:

Pre and Post Session Tracker:

Before the Session:

My Mood is: ☹ ☹ 😐 🙂 😃

How do I feel physically?
(In a scale 1 - 5, with 5 being the best)
☐ ☐ ☐ ☐ ☐

How do I feel emotionally?
(In a scale 1 - 5, with 5 being the best)
☐ ☐ ☐ ☐ ☐

How is the quality of my sleep?
(In a scale 1 - 5, with 5 being the best)
☐ ☐ ☐ ☐ ☐

How was my week in general?
(In a scale 1 - 5, with 5 being the best)
☐ ☐ ☐ ☐ ☐

After the Session:

My Mood is: ☹ ☹ 😐 🙂 😃

Did I feel heard & comfortable?
(In a scale 1 - 5, with 5 being the best)
☐ ☐ ☐ ☐ ☐

How do I feel emotionally now?
(In a scale 1 - 5, with 5 being the best)
☐ ☐ ☐ ☐ ☐

Did this session give me ideas / clarify my thoughts about what to do next?
(In a scale 1 - 5, with 5 being the best)
☐ ☐ ☐ ☐ ☐

How helpful this session was?
(In a scale 1 - 5, with 5 being the best)
☐ ☐ ☐ ☐ ☐

Topic(s) I want to discuss and/or goal(s) my therapist suggested for the session:

(+Optional Reflection ideas: How do I feel about these things / how do they affect my life? Do I already see ways to help myself to get over them?)

Notes from Session: relevant comments & insights.

Reminder: Write here possible actions / "homework" suggested by the therapist

(Complete during or after the session)

The main things that I want to remember from today are:

(Some ideas: Homework, key takeaways, reminders for your next session, challenges to keep in mind and wins to be celebrated!)

- ■
- ■
- ■

Session Date:

Session #:

Next Session Date:

Pre and Post Session Tracker:

Before the Session:	After the Session:

My Mood is: ☹ ☹ 😐 ☺ 😄

My Mood is: ☹ ☹ 😐 ☺ 😄

How do I feel physically?
(In a scale 1 - 5, with 5 being the best)
☐ ☐ ☐ ☐ ☐

Did I feel heard & comfortable?
(In a scale 1 - 5, with 5 being the best)
☐ ☐ ☐ ☐ ☐

How do I feel emotionally?
(In a scale 1 - 5, with 5 being the best)
☐ ☐ ☐ ☐ ☐

How do I feel emotionally now?
(In a scale 1 - 5, with 5 being the best)
☐ ☐ ☐ ☐ ☐

How is the quality of my sleep?
(In a scale 1 - 5, with 5 being the best)
☐ ☐ ☐ ☐ ☐

Did this session give me ideas / clarify my thoughts about what to do next?
(In a scale 1 - 5, with 5 being the best)
☐ ☐ ☐ ☐ ☐

How was my week in general?
(In a scale 1 - 5, with 5 being the best)
☐ ☐ ☐ ☐ ☐

How helpful this session was?
(In a scale 1 - 5, with 5 being the best)
☐ ☐ ☐ ☐ ☐

Topic(s) I want to discuss and/or goal(s) my therapist suggested for the session:

(+Optional Reflection ideas: How do I feel about these things / how do they affect my life? Do I already see ways to help myself to get over them?)

Notes from Session: relevant comments & insights.

Reminder: Write here possible actions / "homework" suggested by the therapist

(Complete during or after the session)

The main things that I want to remember from today are:

(Some ideas: Homework, key takeaways, reminders for your next session, challenges to keep in mind and wins to be celebrated!)

■

■

■

Session Date:

Session #:

Next Session Date:

Pre and Post Session Tracker:

Before the Session:

My Mood is: ☹ ☹ 😐 🙂 😃

How do I feel physically?
(In a scale 1 - 5, with 5 being the best)
☐ ☐ ☐ ☐ ☐

How do I feel emotionally?
(In a scale 1 - 5, with 5 being the best)
☐ ☐ ☐ ☐ ☐

How is the quality of my sleep?
(In a scale 1 - 5, with 5 being the best)
☐ ☐ ☐ ☐ ☐

How was my week in general?
(In a scale 1 - 5, with 5 being the best)
☐ ☐ ☐ ☐ ☐

After the Session:

My Mood is: ☹ ☹ 😐 🙂 😃

Did I feel heard & comfortable?
(In a scale 1 - 5, with 5 being the best)
☐ ☐ ☐ ☐ ☐

How do I feel emotionally now?
(In a scale 1 - 5, with 5 being the best)
☐ ☐ ☐ ☐ ☐

Did this session give me ideas / clarify my thoughts about what to do next?
(In a scale 1 - 5, with 5 being the best)
☐ ☐ ☐ ☐ ☐

How helpful this session was?
(In a scale 1 - 5, with 5 being the best)
☐ ☐ ☐ ☐ ☐

Topic(s) I want to discuss and/or goal(s) my therapist suggested for the session:

(+Optional Reflection ideas: How do I feel about these things / how do they affect my life? Do I already see ways to help myself to get over them?)

Notes from Session: relevant comments & insights.

Reminder: Write here possible actions / "homework" suggested by the therapist

(Complete during or after the session)

The main things that I want to remember from today are:

(Some ideas: Homework, key takeaways, reminders for your next session,
challenges to keep in mind and wins to be celebrated!)

-
-
-

Session Date:

Session #:

Next Session Date:

Pre and Post Session Tracker:

Before the Session:

My Mood is: 😞 😟 😐 🙂 😄

How do I feel physically?
(In a scale 1 - 5, with 5 being the best)
☐ ☐ ☐ ☐ ☐

How do I feel emotionally?
(In a scale 1 - 5, with 5 being the best)
☐ ☐ ☐ ☐ ☐

How is the quality of my sleep?
(In a scale 1 - 5, with 5 being the best)
☐ ☐ ☐ ☐ ☐

How was my week in general?
(In a scale 1 - 5, with 5 being the best)
☐ ☐ ☐ ☐ ☐

After the Session:

My Mood is: 😞 😟 😐 🙂 😄

Did I feel heard & comfortable?
(In a scale 1 - 5, with 5 being the best)
☐ ☐ ☐ ☐ ☐

How do I feel emotionally now?
(In a scale 1 - 5, with 5 being the best)
☐ ☐ ☐ ☐ ☐

**Did this session give me ideas /
clarify my thoughts about what to
do next?**
(In a scale 1 - 5, with 5 being the best)
☐ ☐ ☐ ☐ ☐

How helpful this session was?
(In a scale 1 - 5, with 5 being the best)
☐ ☐ ☐ ☐ ☐

Topic(s) I want to discuss and/or goal(s) my therapist suggested for the session:

(+Optional Reflection ideas: How do I feel about these things / how do they affect my life?
Do I already see ways to help myself to get over them?)

Notes from Session: relevant comments & insights.

Reminder: Write here possible actions / "homework" suggested by the therapist

(Complete during or after the session)

The main things that I want to remember from today are:

(Some ideas: Homework, key takeaways, reminders for your next session, challenges to keep in mind and wins to be celebrated!)

- ◼
- ◼
- ◼

Session Date:

Next Session Date:

Session #:

Pre and Post Session Tracker:

Before the Session:	After the Session:

My Mood is: ☹ 🙁 😐 🙂 😀

How do I feel physically?
(In a scale 1 - 5, with 5 being the best)
☐ ☐ ☐ ☐ ☐

How do I feel emotionally?
(In a scale 1 - 5, with 5 being the best)
☐ ☐ ☐ ☐ ☐

How is the quality of my sleep?
(In a scale 1 - 5, with 5 being the best)
☐ ☐ ☐ ☐ ☐

How was my week in general?
(In a scale 1 - 5, with 5 being the best)
☐ ☐ ☐ ☐ ☐

My Mood is: ☹ 🙁 😐 🙂 😀

Did I feel heard & comfortable?
(In a scale 1 - 5, with 5 being the best)
☐ ☐ ☐ ☐ ☐

How do I feel emotionally now?
(In a scale 1 - 5, with 5 being the best)
☐ ☐ ☐ ☐ ☐

Did this session give me ideas / clarify my thoughts about what to do next?
(In a scale 1 - 5, with 5 being the best)
☐ ☐ ☐ ☐ ☐

How helpful this session was?
(In a scale 1 - 5, with 5 being the best)
☐ ☐ ☐ ☐ ☐

Topic(s) I want to discuss and/or goal(s) my therapist suggested for the session:

(+Optional Reflection ideas: How do I feel about these things / how do they affect my life? Do I already see ways to help myself to get over them?)

Notes from Session: relevant comments & insights.

Reminder: Write here possible actions / "homework" suggested by the therapist

(Complete during or after the session)

The main things that I want to remember from today are:

(Some ideas: Homework, key takeaways, reminders for your next session, challenges to keep in mind and wins to be celebrated!)

- ▪
- ▪
- ▪

Pre and Post Session Tracker:

Before the Session:

My Mood is: ☹ ☹ 😐 🙂 😄

How do I feel physically?
(In a scale 1 - 5, with 5 being the best)
☐ ☐ ☐ ☐ ☐

How do I feel emotionally?
(In a scale 1 - 5, with 5 being the best)
☐ ☐ ☐ ☐ ☐

How is the quality of my sleep?
(In a scale 1 - 5, with 5 being the best)
☐ ☐ ☐ ☐ ☐

How was my week in general?
(In a scale 1 - 5, with 5 being the best)
☐ ☐ ☐ ☐ ☐

After the Session:

My Mood is: ☹ ☹ 😐 🙂 😄

Did I feel heard & comfortable?
(In a scale 1 - 5, with 5 being the best)
☐ ☐ ☐ ☐ ☐

How do I feel emotionally now?
(In a scale 1 - 5, with 5 being the best)
☐ ☐ ☐ ☐ ☐

Did this session give me ideas / clarify my thoughts about what to do next?
(In a scale 1 - 5, with 5 being the best)
☐ ☐ ☐ ☐ ☐

How helpful this session was?
(In a scale 1 - 5, with 5 being the best)
☐ ☐ ☐ ☐ ☐

Topic(s) I want to discuss and/or goal(s) my therapist suggested for the session:

(+Optional Reflection ideas: How do I feel about these things / how do they affect my life? Do I already see ways to help myself to get over them?)

Notes from Session: relevant comments & insights.

Reminder: Write here possible actions / "homework" suggested by the therapist

(Complete during or after the session)

The main things that I want to remember from today are:

(Some ideas: Homework, key takeaways, reminders for your next session, challenges to keep in mind and wins to be celebrated!)

- ■
- ■
- ■

Session Date:

Session #:

Next Session Date:

Pre and Post Session Tracker:

Before the Session:

My Mood is: 😠 😟 😐 🙂 😀

How do I feel physically?
(In a scale 1 - 5, with 5 being the best)
☐ ☐ ☐ ☐ ☐

How do I feel emotionally?
(In a scale 1 - 5, with 5 being the best)
☐ ☐ ☐ ☐ ☐

How is the quality of my sleep?
(In a scale 1 - 5, with 5 being the best)
☐ ☐ ☐ ☐ ☐

How was my week in general?
(In a scale 1 - 5, with 5 being the best)
☐ ☐ ☐ ☐ ☐

After the Session:

My Mood is: 😠 😟 😐 🙂 😀

Did I feel heard & comfortable?
(In a scale 1 - 5, with 5 being the best)
☐ ☐ ☐ ☐ ☐

How do I feel emotionally now?
(In a scale 1 - 5, with 5 being the best)
☐ ☐ ☐ ☐ ☐

Did this session give me ideas / clarify my thoughts about what to do next?
(In a scale 1 - 5, with 5 being the best)
☐ ☐ ☐ ☐ ☐

How helpful this session was?
(In a scale 1 - 5, with 5 being the best)
☐ ☐ ☐ ☐ ☐

Topic(s) I want to discuss and/or goal(s) my therapist suggested for the session:

(+Optional Reflection ideas: How do I feel about these things / how do they affect my life? Do I already see ways to help myself to get over them?)

Notes from Session: relevant comments & insights.

Reminder: Write here possible actions / "homework" suggested by the therapist
(Complete during or after the session)

The main things that I want to remember from today are:

(Some ideas: Homework, key takeaways, reminders for your next session,
challenges to keep in mind and wins to be celebrated!)

-
-
-

Session Date: _____   **Session #:** _____

Next Session Date: _____

Pre and Post Session Tracker:

Before the Session:	After the Session:
My Mood is: ☹ ☹ 😐 🙂 😄	**My Mood is:** ☹ ☹ 😐 🙂 😄
How do I feel physically? (In a scale 1 - 5, with 5 being the best) ▢▢▢▢▢	**Did I feel heard & comfortable?** (In a scale 1 - 5, with 5 being the best) ▢▢▢▢▢
How do I feel emotionally? (In a scale 1 - 5, with 5 being the best) ▢▢▢▢▢	**How do I feel emotionally now?** (In a scale 1 - 5, with 5 being the best) ▢▢▢▢▢
How is the quality of my sleep? (In a scale 1 - 5, with 5 being the best) ▢▢▢▢▢	**Did this session give me ideas / clarify my thoughts about what to do next?** (In a scale 1 - 5, with 5 being the best) ▢▢▢▢▢
How was my week in general? (In a scale 1 - 5, with 5 being the best) ▢▢▢▢▢	**How helpful this session was?** (In a scale 1 - 5, with 5 being the best) ▢▢▢▢▢

Topic(s) I want to discuss and/or goal(s) my therapist suggested for the session:

(+Optional Reflection ideas: How do I feel about these things / how do they affect my life? Do I already see ways to help myself to get over them?)

Notes from Session: relevant comments & insights.

Reminder: Write here possible actions / "homework" suggested by the therapist

(Complete during or after the session)

The main things that I want to remember from today are:

(Some ideas: Homework, key takeaways, reminders for your next session, challenges to keep in mind and wins to be celebrated!)

- ◼
- ◼
- ◼

Session Date:

Session #:

Next Session Date:

Pre and Post Session Tracker:

Before the Session:

My Mood is: 🙁 😦 😐 🙂 😃

How do I feel physically?
(In a scale 1 - 5, with 5 being the best)
☐ ☐ ☐ ☐ ☐

How do I feel emotionally?
(In a scale 1 - 5, with 5 being the best)
☐ ☐ ☐ ☐ ☐

How is the quality of my sleep?
(In a scale 1 - 5, with 5 being the best)
☐ ☐ ☐ ☐ ☐

How was my week in general?
(In a scale 1 - 5, with 5 being the best)
☐ ☐ ☐ ☐ ☐

After the Session:

My Mood is: 🙁 😦 😐 🙂 😃

Did I feel heard & comfortable?
(In a scale 1 - 5, with 5 being the best)
☐ ☐ ☐ ☐ ☐

How do I feel emotionally now?
(In a scale 1 - 5, with 5 being the best)
☐ ☐ ☐ ☐ ☐

Did this session give me ideas / clarify my thoughts about what to do next?
(In a scale 1 - 5, with 5 being the best)
☐ ☐ ☐ ☐ ☐

How helpful this session was?
(In a scale 1 - 5, with 5 being the best)
☐ ☐ ☐ ☐ ☐

Topic(s) I want to discuss and/or goal(s) my therapist suggested for the session:

(+Optional Reflection ideas: How do I feel about these things / how do they affect my life? Do I already see ways to help myself to get over them?)

Notes from Session: relevant comments & insights.

Reminder: Write here possible actions / "homework" suggested by the therapist

(Complete during or after the session)

The main things that I want to remember from today are:

(Some ideas: Homework, key takeaways, reminders for your next session, challenges to keep in mind and wins to be celebrated!)

■

■

■

Session Date:

Session #:

Next Session Date:

Pre and Post Session Tracker:

Before the Session:

My Mood is: ☹ ☹ 😐 🙂 😄

How do I feel physically?
(In a scale 1 - 5, with 5 being the best)
☐ ☐ ☐ ☐ ☐

How do I feel emotionally?
(In a scale 1 - 5, with 5 being the best)
☐ ☐ ☐ ☐ ☐

How is the quality of my sleep?
(In a scale 1 - 5, with 5 being the best)
☐ ☐ ☐ ☐ ☐

How was my week in general?
(In a scale 1 - 5, with 5 being the best)
☐ ☐ ☐ ☐ ☐

After the Session:

My Mood is: ☹ ☹ 😐 🙂 😄

Did I feel heard & comfortable?
(In a scale 1 - 5, with 5 being the best)
☐ ☐ ☐ ☐ ☐

How do I feel emotionally now?
(In a scale 1 - 5, with 5 being the best)
☐ ☐ ☐ ☐ ☐

Did this session give me ideas / clarify my thoughts about what to do next?
(In a scale 1 - 5, with 5 being the best)
☐ ☐ ☐ ☐ ☐

How helpful this session was?
(In a scale 1 - 5, with 5 being the best)
☐ ☐ ☐ ☐ ☐

Topic(s) I want to discuss and/or goal(s) my therapist suggested for the session:

(+Optional Reflection ideas: How do I feel about these things / how do they affect my life? Do I already see ways to help myself to get over them?)

Notes from Session: relevant comments & insights.

Reminder: Write here possible actions / "homework" suggested by the therapist

(Complete during or after the session)

The main things that I want to remember from today are:

(Some ideas: Homework, key takeaways, reminders for your next session, challenges to keep in mind and wins to be celebrated!)

- ▪
- ▪
- ▪

Additional Notes

Suggestions of things to think & write about:

You may use these pages if you need additional space to write during your therapy session. Alternatively, you can use these pages to reflect between sessions:

- How do I feel about these things and how do they affect my life? Do I already see ways to help myself to get over them?

- Try to describe your dreams before and after your therapy session

- Important reminders for my Therapy Sessions (eg. triggers and events events that happened between sessions)

- Challenges to keep in mind

- Small and big wins to be celebrated

November 20, 2021
Conversation with Richard

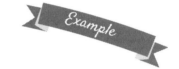

I talked to Richard today and I feel very relieved.

He has been feeling strange about our relationship too and agreed that we needed to talk. He was a bit defensive about spending time alone in the computer (he said that the evenings are his only chance to catch up, since during the day he is at work, and doesn't have access to a computer nor can check his phone very often).

I still don't know what will happen to our relationship over time, but we agreed to watch a movie together once a week, and to try to do more things outdoors, too.

One idea that crossed my mind during our conversation was to propose that we attend therapy sessions together – Marriage / Couples Therapy sessions. But I didn't say that yet. I think he will refuse it. One step at a time.

After this conversation I feel less "paralyzed" and more encouraged to search for a new job. I hope to find at least a seasonal job during the holidays!

Thank you For Using This Journal. We Hope you liked it!

We are on a journey of publishing 52 journals this year!
We would love to invite you to check out one of our other Journals:

Therapy Journals

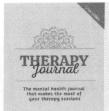

THERAPY JOURNAL:

This is a journal with prompts (questions and suggestions), and it was designed to support you during 30 therapy sessions, no matter how often they take place (ie. it will be ok if you use it twice a week, once a week, or once every 2 weeks). It also includes important recommendations that will help you make the most of your therapy sessions.

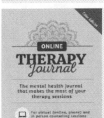

ONLINE THERAPY JOURNAL:

Similar to the above, this is a journal with prompts (questions and suggestions), and it was designed to support you during 30 virtual / telephonic therapy sessions, no matter how often they take place (eg. twice a week, once a week, or once every 2 weeks). The difference it that this journal gives recommendations for VIRTUAL sessions.

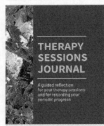

THERAPY SESSIONS JOURNAL:

If you like to write in LINED journals, this is the one for you! This journal also has prompts (questions & suggestions), and it was designed to support you during 6 months of therapy (with weekly therapy sessions, ie. 4-5 sessions per month). This therapy journal will help you make the most of your therapy and self-reflection sessions.!

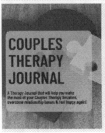

COUPLES THERAPY JOURNAL:

This journal has 3 main spaces for you to write in: (1) a space for you to write what is the focus of each session , (2) a space to capture how your partner is thinking and feeling and what he/she is sharing, (3) and finally a space for you to write your own insights & takeaways during counseling sessions. The right choice for people attending Couples Therapy!

Therapist Journal

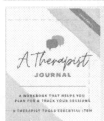

A THERAPIST JOURNAL:

Encouraged and guided by a professional therapist, we created this journal to provide the best help for therapists, both in their preparation for the therapy sessions, and during the sessions themselves.
This journal is what we were told would be the most efficient way for organizing therapist notes, all in one place!

Kids

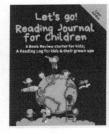

LET'S GO READING JOURNAL FOR CHILDREN:

This journal was created to encourage kids to have reading & discussion time with their grown ups. It also includes key recommendations for the grown ups on how to make the most of reading time with kids. And the "big readers" will have a wonderful record of the child's assisted reading journey.

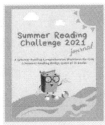

SUMMER READING JOURNAL FOR CHILDREN:

This child-friendly journal will help caregivers and children establish a reading routine during this summer. After going through the challenge of 25 books this summer, kids will learn to look forward to reading & discussion time, and the "big readers" will have a record of the child's reading progress made over time! This journal also includes a list of suggested activities for the summer

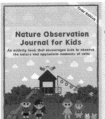

NATURE OBSERVATION JOURNAL FOR CHILDREN:

This "draw and write journal" will encourage you to spend family time in contact with nature, even if you live in a city.
With it you will record your child's nature observations and will encourage him/her to draw what he/she saw, or represent how he/she felt while in contact with nature

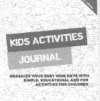

KIDS ACTIVITIES JOURNAL FOR CHILDREN:

This journal was designed with the goal to support families in developing a healthier, more organized and efficient routine of activities while raising their children. It will help you plan for playful activities, games & hobbies with children, in addition to encouraging them to do school work and help with chores.

Motherhood, Fatherhood & Family

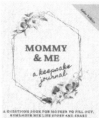

MOMMY & ME
A KEEPSAKE JOURNAL

This is a journal with prompts that will guide a mother to write about her memories and prepare her children to thrive in life by learning mom's important advice & lessons.
Fill any page, at any time, until you complete the journal, or feel that "it's ready". Then give it (back) as a treasured gift to your child!

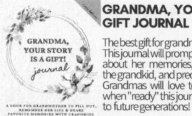

GRANDMA, YOUR STORY IS A GIFT JOURNAL

The best gift for grandma!
This journal will prompt a grandmother to write about her memories, special moments with the grandkid, and precious advice.
Grandmas will love to share their story, and when "ready" this journal will be a treasured gift to future generations!

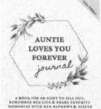

AUNTIE LOVES YOU FOREVER JOURNAL

This is a journal with prompts that will guide an auntie to write about her memories and prepare her nephews & nieces to thrive in life by learning important advice and lessons. Fill any page, at any time, until you complete the journal, or feel that "it's ready". Then give this precious gift (back) to your nephews & nieces!

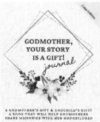

GODMOTHER, YOUR STORY IS A GIFT JOURNAL

A godmother's gift & godchild's gift!
This journal with prompts will guide a godmother to write about her treasured memories and important recommendations that she would like to share with her godchild.
Fill any page, at any time, until you feel that "it's ready" to be gifted to your godchildren.

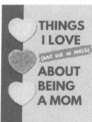

THINGS I LOVE (AND NOT SO MUCH) ABOUT BEING A MOM:

This is a blank / lined journal for moms to write about motherhood experiences – good and bad days – and make the most out of all of their days. It will help you normalize what's normal, feel more relaxed, and clear your mind.
And over time you will have a beautiful collection of "motherhood moments"!

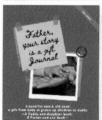

FATHER YOUR STORY IS A GIFT JOURNAL

This is a journal with prompts that will guide a father to write about his memories and prepare his children to thrive in life by learning dad's important advice & lessons.
Fill any page, at any time, until you complete the journal, or feel that "it's ready". Then give it (back) as a treasured gift to your child!

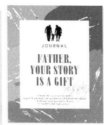

PRIDE VERSION - FATHER, YOUR STORY IS A GIFT

This is a journal with prompts that will guide a LGBTQ father to write about his memories and prepare his children to thrive in life by learning dad's important advice & lessons.
Fill any page, at any time, until you complete the journal, or feel that "it's ready". Then give it (back) as a treasured gift to your child!

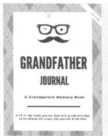

GRANDFATHER JOURNAL.
A GRANDPARENT MEMORY BOOK

The best gift for grandpa!
This journal will prompt a grandfather to write about his memories, special moments with the grandkid, and precious advice.
Grandpas will love to share their story, and when "ready" this journal will be a treasured gift to future generations!

Happiness, Inner Peace, Resilience & Improving Relationships

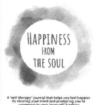

HAPPINESS FROM THE SOUL

This "self-therapy" happiness journal is exactly what you need to start to implement daily 3 things that a Harvard professor teaches : Organize your errands / Message someone important/ Write a journal entry.
After a few days doing this, you're very likely to start feeling happier!

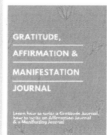

GRATITUDE, AFFIRMATION AND MANIFESTATION JOURNAL

This journal brings it all to you: Gratitude, Affirmation & Manifestation. These habits together can emanate the best feelings within us and help us become calmer and more resilient. They can help us live a happier life and can give us the encouragement to pursue our goals. In summary, this journal will help you relax and connect with the best within you to create the life of your dreams.

... and more!

Check our full collection on Amazon.

★ ★ ★ ★ ★

Journals available in other Languages

Our journals are available on Amazon in English, German, French and Italian (with more languages to come soon).

Join our "Launch Team"

If you would like to to receive free samples of future journals to help us validating concepts, with cover visual selection and more, please let us know!

--> New journals are launched almost every week! <--

Connect with us & Leave your Review on Amazon

**If for any reason you are not satisfied with your journal,
please contact us directly;
we will do our best to make you happy!**

*And, especially if you're happy with the journal,
we'd really appreciate if you could leave an honest review on Amazon
(even just the star rating helps us a lot!)*

**We would love to stay connected, and receive your comments or suggestions.
Follow / message / tag us / leave a review:
- on Amazon: A Day to Remember Journals
- Instagram: @adaytoremember_journals
- OR email: adaytoremember.journals@gmail.com.**

*With much gratitude,
Carla and Milena*

Made in the USA
Columbia, SC
14 December 2024